ROSARY ROAD: My Journey Through Cancer

I had just graduated from Nursing School in 1979 when I, my husband and two young children moved from Chicago Illinois to Houston Texas. My husband was planning to attend the University of Houston to complete a degree plan in Laser-Optic Science. It was the only place in the country he could get a bachelor's degree in this field. It was a bold move for our little family to move from Chicago with the freezing climate to such a humid and tropical environment. Also, to leave the Catholic school system and our Catholic religious practice. Houston had an oil Industry economic base which was very foreign to us. My husband had been going to night school and was, by day, a Chicago policeman. Upon our arrival, we bought a house, my husband started in his scholastic journey at the university, and I was starting my first job as a Registered Nurse. I also had to begin to get our children enrolled in school. This was confusing to me because the Catholic school system was obviously smaller in Houston. Only grades from Kindergarten through fourth grade were available at the Catholic School that was located a few miles down the road from our new house. I was reluctant to enroll them in this Catholic school system in Houston because I knew little of their practice in Texas. We had not been fond of the Catholic School System in Chicago. It was brutal and unforgiving in many social and academic practices. That being said, we thought they had received an acceptable early school education though. The day I was enrolling them in the new Catholic School, when I was filling in the paper work, the TV in the office room started reporting that the current Catholic Pope had been shot. The ladies in the office began to walk over to the TV and stand there in moaning horror, not noticing the moment I fled, to escape their presence, right out the door. I went down the same street, the other way. I enrolled them in the public school system before I lost my nerve. I felt guilty, but inspired. I hoped I had done the right thing for them. I wanted them to experience something more in their lives. I wasn't sure exactly what that was, but I felt a bit driven to do it. It was a bold move by this Catholic girl. I had come through the Catholic School System in Chicago from kindergarten until my eighteenth birthday. Just after I graduated from a girls Catholic High School I married a big hunk of a guy, a Marine Sergeant, who was and still is the love of my life. We married in our local Catholic Church. This is also where we baptized our two children.

Several years later. My husband finished his degree, I advanced in my nursing positions at the local hospital. The kids did great in the public school system eventually graduating and going onto Sam Houston University where they both graduated. We attended the Catholic Church on most Sundays, when we could. Guess we could all call ourselves Catholic and be proud of it. I never could have dreamed what began some of the darkest days of the Catholic Church that no one ever expected. There was so much mystery and unbelievable deceit being constantly uncovered. It seemed it never would end. What did this mean. Religion suddenly seemed so questionable in its meaning. I wanted something rock solid to count on and live my life by. I was on shaky ground finding that with this going on. Did this have some Godly purpose? Had man fouled up the concept of religion and ruined faith finally? The bible says there is a " time" for everything. Was this the time to change religion forever? You know, that concept of believing in what you cannot see but believing it was all worth it and it was a good thing to do. This unveiling deceit in the Catholic church was unbelievable. Where could you find the goodness of God in this. Religion today appears to be a broker dome of relentless contribution. When I was a young nurse I would to try and watch the patients I cared for that died to see if there was anything you could see, like energy, or a spirit leaving, or something. I wanted something to happen, something to see, that could provide some answers to some of these questions. I thought maybe now I had the opportunity to see this happen. Sadly, nothing was visible. I was just left with more questions. I was left of the opinion that there is energy that we do not see or understand, probably flowing around us. Maybe we are all stuck in our moments of" time" as we live, and the moment we die those moments end there and maybe that is where we stay in "time". No new energy has ever been created or lost science says. I believe that we have an endless relationship with the energy and the universe above us. There may be forces of energy that flow around us that keeps us directly linked to that universe. With this in mind, I use to tell my family they were "star stuff".

When I was 50 years old I retired from nursing. I had a severe lumbar spine injury when I was 8 years old and I was starting to need a different life style. I thought it was time to take better care of myself and use the time I had to enjoy that. I was a bit uneasy about leaving nursing as I had worked so hard to get my degree. I identified with nursing for a good part of my life. I wanted to stay healthy and enjoy the changes I was making. I had done all that I wanted to do in nursing and more. I was thrilled to have this time with my husband and my grown children. I could talk with my family any time I wanted, I could read, play on the computer, cook good food for them, swim, see doctors when I needed, and travel. The world was mine for the taking, and my family was my world. I was right back where I started so many years ago. I was not too old and retiring early seemed to be the right thing to do. I was happy. I didn't know it, but It wasn't going to be that easy . I didn't see the big "C" coming. No one ever does.

A few years into my retirement, I had a rib on the right side of my chest suddenly pull loose from my sternum. I thought it was a pulled muscle at first. I put on a support, the pain went away eventually and it didn't feel like I had a problem from it. It took a while before I realized it was a loose rib. I do have a rib hump secondary to the spinal injury. I thought maybe the spinal curves were getting worse. The medical options to fix this have been unacceptable. I figured that it was it was just aging and my spinal injury was maybe getting worse. I started to get a small sore on the right side of my chest, right where the rib had pulled loose . The sore was small and pink. I thought the sore was directly related to the rib rubbing the area. The rib would attach and then pull away again. I had a very hopeless attitude when it came time to get any with any of this in the past. The surgery to help with this was barbaric. The surgery was more cosmetic, and it would not relieve any of the pain. I was doing better taking care of myself, so I thought. Suddenly, I started to get this excruciating pain in my right femur, which I had before. It was pretty horrific. It was intolerable actually. As usual, I thought I just had to get through it. Nothing relieved the pain, just time. I couldn't walk or get out of the bed easily. It started to subsided as it had so many times before. I had done this dance so many times. I had severe pain before and the characteristics of the pain had been changing throughout my life. Some of the things I had to deal with my spine in the past took many months to overcome, but I did it. All I kept thinking was that I would heal up as it I had so many times before. I was not sure if this was different. I realized later that I was actually in so much pain I could never have gotten in a car or walked into an office. I would have had to go in an ambulance to get any help. When I realized this, I couldn't' believe I was that sick. I thought if I could get a little better, not in so much pain, I would go see about the sore and my spine. I felt overwhelmed with the idea. Just a few weeks I thought. The pain was slowly subsiding. How many times do we all have something wrong and then we wait a bit and then we would get better. It was a simple miracle that I could walk and do the things I did, but I did. It was bad, but I always got through it, and life would go on. Would that happen this time I thought. It never stopped me before. I was afraid now something would.

I was slowly getting around, and feeling like I was getting stronger. I got up early one Sunday morning and swung my feet over the side of the bed and started to think about what I would do today. I like to cook in the morning for the day as I got weaker as the day moved on. I thought to get up and make a cake and put bread in the bread machine. I started to brace myself on a small stool by my bedside. As I started to stand up I couldn't feel or control my right leg and then I slowly slid to the floor. I didn't actually feel my leg break, I only saw that it was broken, badly. I called for my husband who was in the study. I tried to look back over my should and saw that the bedroom door was closed and the study, I knew, was on the other side of the house. My daughter was asleep upstairs. I called and called, but no one came. I looked down at my leg and it looked badly twisted. Suddenly, I got very afraid. What if no one came in for a while. What if they never hear me. Then I thought " call louder", and I tried again. Finally, the door opened and there was my guy. I knew I would be ok now. He called for our daughter and she called 911. I went in an ambulance to the hospital. I don't remember much of what happened. I was admitted through the emergency room. They immediately took an ex ray of my leg. I thought I was going right from the emergency room into surgery to get my leg set. Then I found out the surgery wasn't going to happen right then. Everyone kind of disappeared. The ex-ray showed cancer in my right femur. They were getting ready to tell me that. That was the reason my femur broke in two. One doctor came and told me that I had cancer in my femur. He told me that me twice. I guess he figured I didn't hear him. I did hear him, but I couldn't believe him. It was just too shocking. Being a nurse I thought I was going to lose my leg. That wasn't right either. They came to my room after they admitted me to tell me that they would try to put a titanium rod and screws in my leg, if an oncologist would agree to the procedure. In approximately 12 hours, one doctor after the other came into my room and added a new cancer diagnosis. It all amounted to having Stage 4 Breast Cancer. I had cancer in my sternum, right breast and chest wall, right lymph node, upper thoracic spine, lower lumbar spine(right in the injury), right femur, right hip and groin. As my daughter told me later crying," it is everywhere". I felt like I had been hit by a freight train going 100 miles an hour. I couldn't think. I just stared at them and agreed to everything. I was grateful for the help. I was also amazed at their proficiency. My family was there. I looked into their eyes and that said it all. Pain. Wow! I had never seen that in them before.

I had the surgery the next day. They put a titanium rod and screws in my right femur as they had said they would. The surgeon who put the rod in my leg said he designed the rod himself. He told me I was a lucky girl because of that. I couldn't agree more. I was lucky, the doctor who fixed my leg would have been my dream choice. He was on call that night and there he was, thank goodness. You know, the experienced doctor you knew had all the knowledge and experience you needed. I was lucky. I always thought I have been very lucky in my life. While I was there in my drugged state, I thought I overheard a nurse in the nursing station talking about a note left in my chart that a social worker from New York called and said not to transfer me out to a rehabilitation hospital. Like I would get stuck there, and that was not a good thing. I was on a lot of narcotics and I am sure a lot was happening that I kind of imaged or didn't get right. Even so, it was a miracle, as this thought was very instrumental in helping me make a plan of goals to save my life. Everyone was trying to help. I was very quickly transferred to a rehabilitation hospital, in an ambulance, the third day of this ordeal. It was very fast, and I wasn't sure this was the right thing to do. I kept thinking they would keep me and I needed to get out and get treated for the cancer. I would wondered in the days that followed, if I had any more lucky charms in my lucky charm bag. I was so weak, and I hadn't realized how far gone I was. I didn't know if I could come back. I didn't know how to come back. I decided I would work very hard, with lots of pain medication, to get out of the rehabilitation facility in two weeks. That seemed logical as the first thing to do. I had to get out to find out how to deal with the cancer. I knew not to "dally" there anymore than I had to. Stage 4

Breast Cancer is lethal. I knew they would want me to stay for at least three weeks as three weeks would be the normal rehabilitation time Medicare would allow in this facility. I needed the care. After the surgery, I literally couldn't do anything by myself. It was so weird being there. I looked younger than a lot of people there, and I found out I actually was older than a lot of them. It was the first time in my life I felt older. 1 am old, I thought. Does someone or something have to tell you that now you are old or does it happen with age or illness? I never wondered these thoughts before. I figured I would do all that when the time came. I wondered if this was the " time". I found out there that I didn't have a Supplement Insurance Policy and badly needed this now. That meant we had to pay all that Medicare did not pay. That is more than you can realize. One of the Oncologist at the hospital told us we had to get a supplement policy or have cash, or maybe I would need to be referred to the indigent hospital in Houston. I wondered why I had spent so many years of my life taking care of sick people and this would be what I had to deal with when I was sick. Was I going to get thrown out with the bath water? I had tried to get a supplement policy a few years ago, but I live in a state that does not allow you to buy that until you are 65 yrs. old. Even though I was in shock and needed help to breathe, there was no relief from the insurance issues, and the money robbery we all experience trying to get health care. I realized that we should never ignore the issues of what could happen to us if we get sick. The main thing is to get the care you need before you need it. Dying is easy. Living is very hard when you are sick. Much of your future depends on the decisions you can make. These decisions may decide if you live or die. You need different options to choose from when you get sick, especially with cancer. There is so much to choose from. I had Medicare, no supplement policy. I got Part D. I got all this for my husband when he turned 65yrs even though he was still working. The baby boomers have a great opportunity. I realized you cannot think you are healthy and you don't need to pay out the money. It is the way it is. If you are covered with Medicare and have a Supplement policy, it is ultimately cheaper than anything else you can do. It will save your family and you much grief if you do get sick. I just couldn't get there before this happened. I had approximately 10 months before I would turn 65. I applied for supplement during Nov/Dec when you can apply if your birthday is within the next year, and they cannot ask you about your health or base premiums on those issue, or deny you insurance.

I was able to be discharged from the rehabilitation hospital in two weeks. I accomplished that with sheer will and a lot of pain medication. It still seemed so hopeless though. How much money did we need to get me the help that I needed? Every place we checked into for cancer treatment based their acceptance on what insurance you had. I had an appointment with the Oncologist I wanted to see the next week. I was lucky she accepted Medicare only. That appointment seemed so far away. I needed answers and I wanted help. I wasn't sure I would get it though. It was the money thing. I was weak and sad. I didn't want to leave my family. I didn't want to get us in debt. I couldn't accept that my family would give anything to help me get well. I didn't want them to compromise themselves like that. I did not know how to ask that. I had never been weak or tired before. Never like this. A nurse came the very day I got home to go over the basic care necessities with me and my husband. One of them was to get " final papers" signed soon. The nurse scared me. She really didn't talk to me, just my husband while I sat and listened. I guess she was knowledgeable about my future longevity. I guess I don't have a chance, I thought. That wasn't a very nice thing to say I thought. I don't know how to leave them. My husband never left my side. I would have surely died if he was not here with me. All of our dreams were gone. I didn't know how to even begin to say goodbye to them. I couldn't picture a world where I wouldn't be with them. I hadn't loved them enough yet. I haven't seen my grandchildren . A physical therapist was to come to the house 3 times a week. I couldn't walk, pick up anything, do anything by myself. I looked at my husband and wondered what was going to happen to him. How could I ask this from him? How could I get well if I couldn't do anything? His unwavering love could be life saving in itself. I wanted to help, but I couldn't do anything!. These were the big questions that had no answer. How much time did I have?

The following days dragged on slowly. Everything was difficult. This was a new world for us. I needed help with literally everything. I finally saw the cancer doctor a week or so later. You can't get these

appointments with your caretakers very easy. It will take time when you feel you have no time. She was very nice, very warm, gave you no false hope, just fact. I was not curable. Three to six months to live if I did not respond to the anti-hormone drug and monthly shot. The monthly shot cost over 5 thousand dollars a month. This was to give me a chance at some quality of life. My chest sore soared to 4 inches by 4 and a half inches. It was sore and bled all the time. I wasn't feeling very lucky. We got the drugs the doctor ordered on the way home. Mostly everyone was saying I was a bad girl. I was told the cancer had been growing a long time. I wondered how long. Years apparently. Like I should have known something. Mostly drugs were for dulling the pain, which was substantial at this point. I began the long journey to wait and see what comes next . I felt so much guilt. I had an overwhelming feeling that I had done something wrong. What that meant I did not know.
I was on so much pain medication I don't really remember much. Everyone was sad. Not much to say. I could see them escape into their own worlds to try to cope with their fears and helplessness. I was glad they could escape. I wished I could.

The oncologist was patient, but she wanted me to get a PET scan as soon as possible. I had never had one in the hospital. I wanted to get the PET scan as well. I had not been able to get the first PET scan as soon as we needed as the insurance company would not authorize it. It would take a lot of energy, concentration, and research to see how much insurance I had and what it would cover. The insurance companies will almost seem to panic (you might be causing them to lose money) and make decisions(like block your authorizations for exams etc.) about your care, very quickly. It will take some time, many days, before you realize what they have done. I was sitting there waiting patiently to get the ok for the scan, going through the hospital staff. You have to know how to fight for yourself. It took several weeks before I realized that there wasn't going to be any scan if I didn't do something about it. These insurance problems make you feel hopeless and helpless when you are the weakest. I cried and cried on the phone begging them to authorize the PET scan so we could see how much cancer I really had. What is new, I cried over everything these days. Finally, after weeks of being on the medication and seeing the oncologist and getting two shots, the insurance authorized the first PET scan. Just as I was ready to get the scan, the machine broke. You have got to be kidding, I thought. I started to wonder if I was ever meant to get this scan. How much cancer did I have? We needed to have a baseline reading of the cancer. I didn't want to be hopeless. My husband and I had learned a long time ago to live every day as best as we can and take time we need to work on our goals. How would I know if I was getting any better if I didn't get this scan. However, in a few days we went to get the can again, and all went well. Right after the scan was done, they wheeled me out on the balcony steps of the scan trailer. My husband just returned and drove up and got out of the car to pick me up. He looked up at the Scan Technician and said immediately as he walked towards us "Is she going to be alright"? When I saw his face, when he said that, my heart broke in a million pieces. The pain and disbelief was so evident in his eyes and face. It was a face of love. I wondered if the other women saw it too. We all stared quietly at him. I was sure I hadn't loved him enough yet. Not yet. They told him he could pick up the report to take to the oncologist in three days. When he went to get it, they gave him a beautiful box of yummy decorated cupcakes. I was sure then they had noticed. This current scan, several weeks later, showed some improvement since the initial cancer levels in the hospital. We now had a baseline to work from. We had flicker of hope. Was this one of those things that teases you and then you fall off the cliff? A cancer diagnosis is such a merry go round. Like you had to carry around a box of chocolates with you and you never knew which one you would get. Everyone tells you the worst that can happen, then hopes tries to cure you, all the while preparing for the worse. All of this screamed that I have to make my own comprehensive plan. I feared getting lost in my own weakness in this mire.

I kept wondering how I could try to fight cancer. Does anyone really know? I was a nurse. I believed you had to have a holistic approach to keeping yourself healthy. A balanced approach to fight disease. I thought patience was part of that. I knew how to do that. This was different. How do you talk to your body? Where is the place you go to heal from within. Where is the starting point? How could you find a center inside yourself to start. I couldn't' do anything, and that includes concentrate on a thought for more than a few seconds. I was home watching Queen Latifah in her new TV program. I would basically get in one place and stay there most of the day. She had an author on that day. She was talking with him about his new book and she mentioned a chapter he devoted to his meditation technique . She had tried it the night before, after reading his book, She really felt herself calmed down from her hectic day. You could imagine that her days were really hectic. She acted like she was really surprised that meditation had helped and that she really liked it. They talked as if you could use anything you wanted to do the actual meditation. The idea was that would concentrate on the meditation. What you used to do it or how you structured it was not so important. Just do it. I thought I remembered that the DaliLama said the same thing. That struck an idea in my head. I had been trying to think or picture what I needed to get myself centered to begin this fight ahead of me. When they were talking, it struck me this was what I needed to try to do. Maybe meditation would help me to concentrate better and calm me down enough to think better. I wanted to make a plan to get well. I remembered that I had a red stoned rosary that my husband and I bought when we went to Rome and toured the Vatican some years back. We bought it after it was blessed by the Pope Paul II. We had seen him in the closed area of the Vatican. I thought, I am a Catholic, I have my own rosary. I know how to use it. It is a meditation piece basically, I thought. Why not use that. What is different. Just the words and the use of the stones to count? Well, I couldn't keep a thought in my head long enough to wonder about it. I was so full of medication effect, anxiety and fear. My once low Blood Pressure was sky high and dangerous. There was nothing I tried helped it get lower. I remembered seeing patients who had cancer when I was working in private practice for several years with a psychiatrist. I never understood why cancer patients were not on drugs to calm them or improved their mood. It was striking. I always thought we humans have a holistic complexity we need to address with treatment. The holistic complex should include: using diet changes , daily vitamins in specific doses to fight disease, foods to fight disease, and exercise to streghthen my body. I reasoned, this plan could decrease the anxiety, and high blood pressure. I felt strongly that I needed something to help me have a fighting chance, not just to have a better quality of life until I died. I couldn't breathe, like I was holding my breath waiting for something. My husband got out our machine that helps you to breathe correctly. We have used it on and off a lot. It really does help to remind you to breathe" right". Will I get better or die? I wanted to try to get better. Maybe this was just the thing to start. I had to start somewhere. I felt optimistic. I was starting to have a plan. Who knew, the Catholic Church had such a great thing here. Say the rosary, my goodness. Maybe this could help me center myself. It was the first time I started to feel maybe I could hope to do something and not just sit here. I went to look for the rosary, and got another idea to also get my great grandmothers beautiful statue of Mary and Jesus. Jesus is supporting Mary with his arm around her, like they are praying together. It is a white porcelain piece with blue and gold roses and a blue rose over Jesus's heart. She used it to burn incense during her life. There is a part in the back of the statue that hold the incense sticks. I shined the silver cross on the rosary and washed the red rosary beads. I put the rosary on the statue and made a plan to get up early and sit and say the rosary before anyone gets up.

Before this happened to me, I had become mostly agnostic. I got up the next morning, and got ready to start saying the rosary. I was thinking I couldn't come to terms or find any peace with any religion. What was I doing with this rosary. I couldn't remember all the prayers. It was beautiful though. I loved the rosary and my Great Grandmothers statue. I found great peace and comfort in these hundred year old things of hers. So many people and family were saying they would pray for me. I didn't know how to think of all this. As a young child I loved to go to church. I believed in things I could not see, I had faith. Manmade religions have become for profit organizations in our time. How did they convince us this was the only way to get what we want. What is it we want? I want to believe in something that enriches my life and not something that enriches them. People do horrible things in the name of religions. Maybe the real miracle is us. The miracle of doing the right thing for each other and ourselves in some kind of harmony. I needed to find a way to calm down and breathe. I needed hope that I could find a way to get well. A lot to ask. I decided to hold the cross and start out by saying that I forgive the people that hurt me in my life and also ask forgiveness for the people that I have hurt. I wondered if these hurts make negative energies

that could take energy away from healing. I wanted to start healing and I believed this was a good place to start. I wanted to get off the ladder of regrets. I believe we start on this ladder very young in our life. We don't even know we are on ,it or give our consent to think this way and do this to ourselves. It is healing and liberating to forgive yourself and others. I then started to advance by saying the rosary like I had been taught. I tried to concentrate and tried to get in touch with my own energy channel. It is said that we are part of the stars. That is where we came from. Kind of one and the same. So I decided to start there. So, if we are linked in this way, I will picture a channel of energy coming into me from above as I say my rosary. I also wanted to picture Mary, Jesus and Pope Pius !! opening the door in the cosmos.
I wondered if these great people are stuck in time with their own energy and are still with us in this way. I want to believe that we each have our own stream of life energy. That we are creating our own life and we will always be on the continuem of time. I wanted to capture that energy source and tap into the strength of it. Every morning, I began my day with this process. I tried not to make it hard to do. Just the best that I could do. It began to be the most important part of the day for me. This was not the only thing I did though.

I also believe in what we call western medicine. I did exactly what the doctors told me to do. I kept every appointment with them religiously with the help of my husband. They told me they could not cure me. I listened. I did not want to believe that I had no power or ability to help myself though. I knew they were pretty smart people. I knew I had choices in everything including who I chose as my doctor, what treatment I wanted and needed. But then I took their lead. I knew I couldn't just decide to try to get well. I had to put a plan in place to do it. I had that choice. I began to put some great effort into what I ate. Cancer loves sugar. You will hear that over and over. What do you do with that information? The more fat you eat, the more sugar you have in your bloodstream and the longer it stays there feeding cancer cells. We have all seen the chubby people on TV, eating fat foods and then tell you to take the pill and then you can eat what you want, no problem. But, if you eat a pizza, for instance, the high fat content will keep the sugar in your blood stream for eight hours before your body can metabolize the fat content and get rid of the sugar in your bloodstream. Logic says maybe I should eat less fat and keep the sugar content down in my diet. We are all supposed to eat several helpings of fruit and vegetables every day. What a chore. All of these items are quickly perishable. How do I buy it and how do I store it. Run to the store every couple of days? I can't ask more of my husband. I can't even go to the bathroom alone. I wondered how I was going to attempt this. It felt daunting.

I decided to get as much of the fruit and vegetables as we could in frozen bags. We had to shop around to find what we wanted. Fruits are easy to buy frozen. Vegetables are much more difficult. I got bags of basic berries. I got a bag strawberries and several apples and vanilla yogurt and honey and a scoop of Vanilla Whey. Then a bag of mixed vegetables with broccoli, cauliflower and carrots, also a bag of frozen spinach. Also a bag of frozen kale. I bought a jar of beets. I got two quarts of V8 juice. Don't add any more vegetables or fruits to these mixtures if you try it. Don't add any of the food that you would not eat right out of the ground. Don't put anything you have to cook to eat in the drink. I use a NUTRiBullet as It mixes the food completely with no clumps, and it is ready to drink easily. A regular blender will not mix this and it will blow up and ruin a blender. You may find another one that does, but approach it in this mindset. Here is how I did it: in the morning, I mixed a few berries and strawberries, a tbsp. of vanilla yogurt, tsp. of honey, two pieces of an apple, scoop of vanilla whey, fill the rest of the beaker up to the line with organic milk. Around three pm every day, I mix about a half of cup of vegetables with broccoli, cauliflower and carrots, spinach, two round small beets, kale, some Mc Cormicks vegetable flavoring, salt and pepper, and fill up to the line on the beaker with V8 juice. I add this all together and the taste is very good. Mix half of the beaker with fruits or vegetables and half with the liquid. If it is too thick and hard to drink then decrease the veggies or fruit until it is ok to drink. I was tempted to put a lot of the fruits and vegetable in the beaker. I realized you can't drink it if you do. It is way too thick. We only eat any regular meals in between these drinks with a mixture of a protein (meat serving 10 oz.), vegetable, and fruit for each meal. Just use one helping of each. Keep the amount of food small as you put it in the beaker. I had to accept that there is only one way to get these drinks so you can make them and you will be able to drink it. After drinking these drinks every day, I could see dramatic improvement in my health. It will be enough for your health to just add small amount of these foods into the drinks each time and then fill with the liquid for each one. I buy frozen fruit and veggies so they last a long time doing this. It is surprising how many drinks you can get out of these bags of frozen fruits and vegetables .

We also take 1000Micro Units B12, 1200 Calcium, 10,000 Units D3 every day. Also Resveratrol 250mg, Multivitamin, Vitamin C 1000 , Aspirin 81mg. , CQ10, Probiotics, and Protandim 1 Tablet . We take these with our morning fruit drink. Because I have breast cancer and it is hormone related, I am trying to limit my exposure to hormones in foods in my diet. Hormone imbalance have a direct link in many cancers. They basically rule our emotional and physical lives in a microcosmic way. One great source of hormone problems I am trying to get away from is milk products. I buy only organic milk. I mix one quart (packet) of powdered milk mixed (I use HEB powdered milk) with water and a quart of organic milk. We like half and half with our coffee so we mix one cup heavy organic cream with our milk mixture or organic milk. We make our own butter with organic heavy cream in a Country Kitchen machine. We make our own ice cream with the same mixtures in a Cuisinart Ice Cream Maker. This is my meager attempt to try to tolerate, and afford, and do as much as I can. For snacks, we would eat the ice cream, piece of cake or a donut. We limit these by serving amount.

At first not too much happened. I started to think of things slowly. I tried to think what to do or what it would take to have a positive outcome. I tried to think of things to get well and get my life, a life with my family back. Getting well is quite a journey. It doesn't just happen. I tried to use the negative energy of the cancer illness and find a way to begin creating positive energy to heal myself. They say, you are what you think. Then my goal is to create a positive life outcome. I didn't expect anything, I just kept the schedule and did the plan. I just hoped it would help. I would try to say the rosary every morning. I was remembering more how to do it. I tried to say it on the way to get the treatment shot every month. It was so hard to concentrate going to a cancer treatment office. I was getting just a shot that hurt, while all the other people in the room were getting chemotherapy. I felt like a big baby compared to the strength and courage I saw in them. My heart bled for them. It was too late for me to get that help, or was I the lucky one to not have it and what if I did get well. These questions would swirl in my head. What if I can get a shot once a month and take a pill every day and really get well. Wouldn't that be something. How many of them would die, like my baby brother was? He was diagnosed with esophageal cancer stage 3 just before me. Would I die or will he? I believe in many energies and forces which are beyond our control and knowledge. I thought if I could get my thinking calmed down and get myself centered in my goals that would be enough. I would be so grateful. I had to learn how to breathe again. As the days continued, I was starting to calm down. I started to feel calm, and kind of happy.

The wound on my chest started to get smaller. It was really noticeable. Then it started to heal faster and faster. It would scab over and fall off and scab over again. Suddenly, my blood work reports were perfect except my salt level was up a little. The doctor was amazed and so were we. She didn't want to change anything because obviously I was responding in a way that surprised her and us. She said to come back in three months, which was also shocking as I had been coming in every 4 weeks. She wanted me to have a PET Scan 3 days before we came in in three months and to get blood work too. I was feeling better. My mind was clearing. I was still weak. I was still having a hard time tolerating too much activity. Walking was getting easier. I kept taking my medication, trying to decrease pain medication and pushing my activity level and, of course, saying my rosary. We bought bikes, I got a three wheeler.

Then something profound happened. I was watching TV and I heard that Pope Paul II was to be canonized a saint. I thought, oh my God, He blessed my rosary, he healed two women of serious illness. I wondered, why not me. I decided to ask Saint Paul to help me get well. I got the news that my baby brother just died of cancer of the esophagus. He was a stage 3, I wondered why he died and I was a stage 4, and I was getting better. A few days after he died, I was just almost awake and I heard his loud deep boisterous voice say my name and say, "everything was going to be okay". I was glad that happened, however it happened. He didn't sound unhappy. I was glad for that. I loved my baby brother.

I will miss him terribly. How can you heal your body without your spirit? I asked Saint Paul to heal me. I kept saying my rosary every day. I went for the PET Scan 3 days before we were to see the Oncologist. The three months were up. I had a lot of trepidation about getting the scan results. I knew the cancer could have spread or it may not have shown on the last scan yet and more would be there now. It may be worse and I may need chemotherapy and radiation to try to rescue me, and or, maybe it will be just too late. Who wants to go get a scan and then see a cancer doctor to tell you the results. The first clue I might be getting a good report was when the lab technician at the PET scan facility called us in the back room to ask where the cancer was in me as we looked at the scan itself. What a strange question to ask me I thought. How could I have Stage Four Breast Cancer and be asked a question like that. I felt like that was very hopeful, but I was kind of in shock and it didn't get in. You have to go and do it though, no choice really. There we sat three days later. It was like being on death row and waiting for the Governor to call to say you would live or die. We waited until she read from her computer, " Well, your labs are perfect", "there is no cancer in your leg, no cancer in your lymph gland, no cancer in your spine, there is a lesion where it started in your chest, but much smaller and at 40% of the intensity than it was, and one small lesion on the head of your femur and at an almost no intensity level, "well, you don't need any chemotherapy or radiation therapy." The lesion on my chest was less than one inch by less than one inch then. I walked in there on my own and my mind was pretty clear. She told me she thinks I am going to be okay. We all kind of sat there staring for a few minutes. It was a bit surreal. Did she say what we thought she said? She, and us, were obviously shocked. She said she didn't want to change anything. I didn't mention the rosary or the diet or exercise. She wanted to see me again in six months. She said I had this for a long time and it would take a long time to go completely away as well. Has the rosary, the food, the love and support healed me? Clearly something was going on here. There is no end to the goodness flowing into my life since this all started. The scan and blood test and the obvious healing were remarkable.

After several months from the date of surgery of getting the rod in my leg, I had an appointment to see the orthopedic surgeon who did the surgery on my leg He is truly remarkable. I have had no pain and I can walk normally, and there is a barely visible scar on my leg from the surgery. The ex-ray of my leg showed a completely healed femur bone with no break or cancer lesions. It was a beautiful bone. He told me they put the rod in my leg to help me "stand a little". The doctors did not expect to see my leg heal. He said this was a miracle. What is a miracle? I was not going to argue with him about that. I'll take it. Strange to have so much cancer and keep hearing that it is gone from these amazing people. We left him again feeling this is so surreal. I am going to see him again in a year. I couldn't believe I am starting to plan months and a year out for things. I will have to see a spine surgeon next. Cancer eats at your healthy cells. It destroys them. When you heal, new cells have to grow. You don't hear much about that. But it is a lot of work for your body to do. I do not know what I will be left to do as I heal. I know my diet will be important for a long time. I will keep saying my rosary every morning. Who knew this Catholic practice of saying the rosary could be put to such beautiful use. All of this is truly remarkable. I can't think of it any other way. Everything changed when I started to pray with my rosary to meditate and bring these changes in my daily life. I believe in the miracle of life. I want to continue to walk on the bridge of time. If you picture that we have the bridge of time that extends back to the beginning of our cosmos, then we all have lots of time, for ages to come. I still have my bag of lucky charms. It is what it is. There will be more to this story I know. It is a year now since I was diagnosed, that I end this story. The next Oncology visit will be around Christmas 2014. I am not ready to have my final time stamp. I am thankful for the time I have to love my husband and my children, and to savor the world around me.

www.ingramcontent.com/pod-product-compliance
Lightning Source LLC
Chambersburg PA
CBHW051422170526
45165CB00004BA/1930